# The Lazy Man's Guide To

# Weight Loss

By J. C. Burns

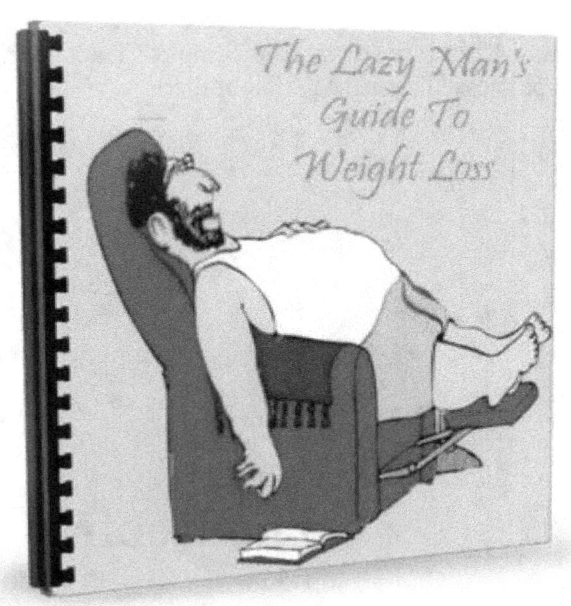

## Preface

First, I would like to make it perfectly clear that I am not a weight loss guru, and I am not a doctor. This is a book from a guy who sits on his butt 10 to 14 hours per day making a living on the internet.

That being said, I would encourage you to check out anything and everything I say here with your doctor, (I think I have to say that, but it's true.) You may have conditions that cannot support what I am telling you here, so please make sure before you start this, (or any other diet program,) that it is safe for your particular body. There is nothing in here to my knowledge that would harm anyone, but by all means, let's be safe. I think I also need to include that results may not be typical. Our bodies are all different, so my results may not be your results. Okay I think I've appeased my attorney.

In any event the choice to better your health is a major one and shouldnt be taken lightly. Give yourself a pat on the back you made the first choice to improve yourself. This book will show you how I was able to get down to respectable weight without exerting extra effort. I hope you enjoy and please read as many times as you need to better yourself.

You have heard the phrase, "Stupid Simple," I am sure. That is what this is. Stupid simple, and painless. That is MY kind of diet!

So...Let's Go!

# The Rebirth
(Mindset is Everything)

At 30, my metabolism has started to slow down, as it does for most people as you grow. It is a natural thing, but it doesn't have to be that way....or at least to the extent that we have taught our bodies to react as we grow older. For many of us, it is an excuse. Laziness and inactivity creeps (especially since the pandemic) into our lives, so we must do something to combat that very thing.

ANY weight loss regimen begins with **YOU**. You must decide in your mind first that you will continue on your weight loss journey no matter how hard because you want the end result. If you don't decide right now to change your habits, your actions, your thoughts then you are doomed from the start. You must take action, *ACTION* is the key word. Nobody can do this for you. You must decide that you are going to change your eating habits. You must decide if you want to be able to start breathing normally again, and start regaining the energy that you have lost.

If you tell yourself that you will not be able to do this, then you won't. You will be stuck saying phrases like "it's too hard or i can't" which is untrue. You have to start with a positive mindset. You have to believe you can do anything you put your mind to. Just knowing that you're doing something that is life changing.

You have to learn to control your mind. It's really a mind game. The mind will play tricks on you to make you feel like you are hungry when you are not. The stomach pains aren't as real as we think. We trick ourselves using time and our mind. We look at the clock and say it's 1 o'clock and I haven't eaten lunch yet even though we had that big breakfast and we aren't even hungry. We still force ourselves to eat that lunch when the body hasn't even finished processing our breakfast yet.

Being able to once again play basketball when at one point I remember being almost 500 lbs and could barely walk up the steps without tiring was life changing for me. Nowadays, my pants fit again, and my belly doesn't hang over my belt the way it used to, I can run up and down the basketball court at any given moment. All of this has given me a new outlook on life. It's a fresh restart, a new beginning.

Never sell yourself short. Believe in yourself, it may sound corny but don't stop believing. Have faith, stick to the plan. You are choosing to do the right thing for your body,mind,spirit, and soul. I am not going to go any further into it, because you have probably already heard it all before. You have probably already beat yourself up enough about it as well. I don't have to tell you about the benefits of losing weight. And I don't have to tell you what diseases are prevalent with people who are obese. These are all common knowledge.

Now your choice is clear and your mind is in a new positive state. Thinking thin is not going to be enough to win the battle, but it is half the battle. Knowing you are taking the steps to improve your life is priceless!

# Dieting and Exercise
(The two word People Hate)

Many, if not all of the weight loss experts, will tell you that exercise and diet must go together. The main reason is that muscle burns fat faster than fat burns fat. Does that make sense? Many people, like myself, really do not have the time, nor the energy (until you lose the pounds,) nor even the inclination to exercise, but because it helps by leaps and bounds to keep your muscles toned, and burn fat, I started doing simple calisthenic or isometric exercises such as jumping jacks, lounges or jogging in place.

An isometric exercise is to tighten your muscles and hold the position for about 10 to 15 seconds, and then let off. It is popular because it took no equipment, and you didn't have to join a gym. Calisthenics are great exercises to help with staying in shape during quarantine. You choose a group of muscles, let's take for example your stomach muscles, or abs. Do 7-10 sit ups, then again 3 or 4 times and that is called a set. You want to remember to breathe. A lot of people tend to hold their breath as they are doing the exercises, which can do you more harm than good. Not only does proper breathing support the exertion of the exercise, but not breathing properly can lead to hernias, exercise induced asthma and a myriad of other life long effects, so please remember to **breathe**.

Your arms can be exercised in the same way. Because each arm has several muscle groups, it is important to rotate your hands for each exercise. Let's do one right now as an example. Start by flexing your bicep and forearm, and then gently rotate your hand and wrist back and forth. Can you feel the different muscle groups? Now do the exercise one arm at a time, and with your hand in 3 different positions for 3 separate exercises. Hold them for 15 seconds, remembering to breathe, then relax them for 30 seconds. Push ups, pull ups and dips are great exercises for beginners, because not only does it work your arm it works your core which is where a lot of your strength comes from.

The legs work the same way. Clenching your thigh muscles for 15 seconds, and relaxing for 30 seconds. Again, 3 sets. Your calf muscles work much in the same way, only you will want to kind of stand on your toes while sitting for 3- 4 sets. You can, and should do  this for your buttocks as well. You will not be "bulking up" during this process, but it will start helping you to tone your muscles, which will begin your weight loss regimen.Squats, glute bridges, and lunges are also great leg workouts for calisthenics. Many athletes and trainers use these workouts to get stronger day to day.

As you begin to lose weight, you are going to want to do more. You will feel the energy again, coursing through your veins and it will propel you to do more. Feeling that energy again is an amazing feeling. The more you do this, the more weight you will lose, and the more energy you are going to have to possibly venture into doing walking, or stair stepping, other cardio exercises or even weighted exercises. Believe me, I do not like to exercise, but the energy I have felt from losing so much weight compels me to keep exercising because I want to continue to feel great.

While some people use weights in their workouts, I have found that any weight works well, including cans of soup. It gives just a little bit more of a resistance to your workout.

I am going to repeat this. We do these exercises to help us burn fat. It will speed your process expeditiously. Honestly, I didn't start using these exercises until I had already lost my initial 15 pounds, which we will be going into in the next phase of the plan.

The thing that triggered my interest in weight loss, was one day I remember coughing up blood in a Red lobster while on a date. SMH! I was never really big but one year i worked for mcdoanlds and i gained 100 lbs in 6 months. I started off not really eating fast food. After a month of working there and learning how to cook the food and make the milkshakes, cookies and fries, I was a pro. At the end of the day I was taking home bags of food. I was making my own sandwiches triple and quadruple burgers, different types of sauces i would put on my burger such as MAC sauce and bbq sauce, stacked up fish sandwiches with extra salt, milkshakes with extra chocolate and a side cone with a huge slab of chocolate drizzled on top. My favorite was the rolo milkshake. I would top it with extra peanut butter cups and chocolate, sprinkles the works. The end result was I had gained an incredible amount of weight in a short time. I went from 230 lbs to 430 lbs in a year or so.

Things that used to be easy became difficult for me. I was much more tired than usual. I stayed in bed for longer periods of time. I watched crazy amounts of tv. I ate huge bowls of cereal and ice cream. I ate cake after cake after cake. I felt as if either i couldn't get full or i would be ready to eat again in ten minutes after I ate.

I remember going to the hospital and the doctor saying all the weight sits on your chest. You will need to lose some weight. From there the doctor put me on a strict regimen that included nothing fried but the food i was allowed to eat i noticed kept me nourished all day and well fed throughout the day. I didn't need to get that candy bar or treat like I used to feel I needed to keep going daily. This was my time and my time to change for good, and so I recollected an article that I had read about the benefits of warm water.

This was the catalyst for my success. I replaced my morning iced tea with water. It was no easy task, as I love my ice tea, but I immediately started feeling better. I didn't get my usual morning jitters from too much sugar, and I seemed to have a bit more energy. I thought that it just might have been in my mind, but it was, in fact, doing something positive to my body. These changes were just the start.

The following pages will describe exactly what I did to lose this weight, and have been able to keep it off, which has been a huge struggle for many including myself.

Aside from drinking water, room temperature more than cold, my eating habits changed as well. This may be the time that you may have problems also. Usually the first couple days to a couple weeks is hard to change at first. I usually didn't eat 1 breakfast but I ate 2. I got up early and cooked breakfast for myself and then got one when I left the house. I started to make myself only eat breakfast off of the plan my doctor gave to me. I incorporated nuts, veggies, fruits, food that were high amounts of protein to keep me filled. I ate oatmeal and a slice of toast, which filled me up perfectly until lunch. If it wasn't oatmeal, and I couldn't get a high protein breakfast, I kept cashews in my pocket if I got hungry before lunch.

Eating the same thing day in and day out gets monotonous, and I really wanted to get those pounds off, so the variety was welcomed. The key here is to not let yourself get bored with what you eat. Eggs once or twice a week is a good start. The importance of breakfast should not be overlooked. You need to eat to lose weight, believe it or not. If I got hungry between lunch and dinner, I would grab an apple or a banana. I was not willing to clog myself up with any other kinds of things for a snack.

The trick here is to not let yourself get hungry. You must eat to keep up your metabolism. The diets where you starve yourself can do real damage to your body. Your body will actually cannibalize itself, by stealing essential  nutrients from your organs and muscles, to satisfy its requirements in less important areas. You may lose weight, but most times you will gain it back in a very short period and it is bad for the rest of your body, especially your organs like the heart and brain.

Snacks between meals are important, as long as it's the right thing to eat. Like I said, fresh fruit, (not canned), and fresh vegetables are the best. Nuts such as cashews are very helpful as well. I don't think I have to say this, but cookies, candy, gummies will only slow your progress.

The other thing we have to give up on this journey is fast food. NO diet has any chance at all if you continue to stop by McDonalds or Burger King for a "snack".  If you are serious about losing weight, fast food joints should go away from your life completely. When you have completed your goal, give thanks and go treat yourself to a small fry, maybe a burger. You've earned that right, but **DON'T** make it a habit.

# Sugary Drinks vs. Water

For some its soda, others its coffee, as for me, it was Ice tea or sweet tea to be exact. I had no idea that a simple iced tea was actually hindering my weight loss goals. Again, I didn't find this out until I was curious one day and looked it up. This was long after I started losing the pounds. Less of the ice tea because plain iced tea is good for you. But the sugar in sweet tea is not.

I want to include this article by Joe Leech, which helps explain the effects of sugary drinks on your body. In which, he lists 13 reasons sugar is not good for you.

"When consumed in excess, added sugar can adversely affect your health However, some sources of sugar are worse than others — and sugary drinks are by far the worst. This primarily applies to sugary soda but also to fruit juices, highly sweetened coffees, and other sources of liquid sugar."

Ive learned throughout the years that the body can survive off of water alone for many days without eating. That is actually how the body works at optimal capacity. Not eating everyday allows the stomach to break down and process the food properly for the body. Everyone has heard the saying our body is made of 70% water, well that is slightly untrue. Our body is actually made of H2O3 which is actually only found in fruit. Fruit and water is really the only source we need to put in our body to run at the peak capacity that we need it to.

Quickly, I do have an online health course coming out on Teachable called Mind, Body and Soul. That will expand deeper into what I said in my previous paragraph. It will also include my 40 day cleanse diet, how to get healthier products to use on our bodies because what we use on our bodies is absorbed through the skin into our system. How to work on controlling our minds from trickery, and much more. I urge you to check it out. It will be fully published online by January 2023.

# Coffee

I had no idea that coffee could hinder weight loss goals. Again, I didn't find this out until I was curious, during my initial weight loss journey and looked it up. This was long after I started losing the pounds.

I want to include this article by James Bowden, which helps explain the effects of coffee on your body.

*I myself am not a coffee drinker but i know many people that had many battles with Starbucks. It's a difficult habit to break. I can tell you this, from the experience of others: When you break the coffee habit, you will feel your own power and energy and be in touch with your own natural energetic rhythms. You may even find that a caffeine-free existence is a great boost to your weight-loss efforts.*

*Although I am not be ready to say that something as basic to American life as coffee is a "drug," we can certainly say that it has drug-like properties:*

*It's addictive.*

*It's a stimulant.*

*It alters mood.*

*There are two basic reasons coffee is a problem for the person trying to lose weight. (It's no bargain for the person who isn't either, by the way). The first reason is psychological, the second physiological.*

*Coffee fits neatly into the receptors for a brain chemical known as adenosine, which is partly responsible for calming you down. By interrupting the activity of adenosine, coffee makes you feel awake and wired. You may think that's a good thing, but consider that virtually every study of PMS has implicated caffeine as a major culprit. The added stimulation and nervousness from the coffee makes you feel edgy at exactly the time that feeling calm would be a blessing. And the blood sugar fluctuations it produces contributes enormously to cravings.*

*Coffee is socially connected to rituals that involve eating. Many of these eating rituals, in turn, are connected to snacks and breaks, fast-food breakfasts and desserts. (Notice that the first beverage you think of when asked what you want with your "Dunkin' Donuts" is not green tea or water.)*

*Coffee stimulates the adrenals, the glands responsible for stress hormones. The constant assault on these poor glands, from coffee, sugar, stress and daily life, can ultimately lead to a condition known as adrenal exhaustion.*

*Coffee plays havoc with your blood sugar. The body treats a coffee jolt as a "stress response" much like the adrenals shooting a jolt of adrenaline into the system. This adrenaline response was a survival mechanism for our caveman ancestors; it signaled danger from a wooly mammoth and told the body to prepare for fight or flight. It signaled the body to release sugar into the blood, to be used as fuel for the muscles (which would be either clubbing that mammoth or climbing the nearest tree). But nowadays, it just signals the release of sugar. With no ensuing flight or flight, the sugar signals a release of insulin, and before you know it, after a couple of hours of jitteriness, your blood sugar is in the toilet, and you're crashing and burning and reaching for ... guess what? I'll give you a hint: It's not Brussels sprouts and steak.*

*Coffee also increases urinary secretion of important minerals such as magnesium, potassium and sodium and uses up a fair amount of vitamin B1. Not only that, the coffee plant itself is a virtual repository for toxins such as pesticides and other harmful chemicals. (If you still insist on drinking it after reading this article, consider buying organic). And it can raise blood pressure and interfere with sleep.*

*Although in the short run it may suppress appetite, over the course of a day most people find it stimulates cravings more than suppresses them.*

*If you are "running on empty," getting your "energy" from artificial stimulants like caffeine, you never really get to understand the effect your food is having on you. You never know whether your food is producing energy and alertness or tiredness and fatigue. You're masking the effects of your eating style with an overpowering stimulant. And that's keeping you from valuable knowledge about what foods work for you and what foods you ought to stay away from.*

There is a myth that coffee and green tea have the same amount of calories. Nothing could be further from the truth.

The average cup of coffee can have anywhere from 80-175 mg of caffeine, depending on the method of preparation. By comparison, the average cup of green tea has about 25-30mg of caffeine.

Furthermore, green tea has a number of health benefits (preventing cancer, battling diabetes, fighting cholesterol, boosting the immune system...) and it is recommended to drink 4-5 cups each day to reap the full benefits. According to researchers, it's safe to drink up 10 cups of green tea a day.

# 1. Sugary Drinks Do Not Make You Feel Full and Are Strongly Linked to Weight Gain

The most common form of added sugar — sucrose or table sugar — supplies large amounts Fructose does not lower the hunger hormone ghrelin or stimulate fullness in the same way as glucose, the sugar that forms when you digest starchy foods.Thus, when you consume liquid sugar, you usually add it on top of your total calorie intake — because sugary drinks don't make you feel full.In one study, people who drank sugary soda in addition to their current diet consumed 17% more calories than before.Not surprisingly, studies show that people who drink sugar-sweetened beverages consistently gain more weight than people who don't.In one study in children, each daily serving of sugar-sweetened beverages was linked to a 60% increased risk of obesity.In fact, sugary drinks are among the most fattening aspects of the modern diet.

# 2. Large Amounts of Sugar Are Turned into Fat in Your Liver

Sucrose or commonly known as sugar and high-fructose corn syrup are composed of two molecules — glucose and fructose — in almost equal amounts. Glucose can be metabolized by every cell in your body, whereas fructose can only be metabolized by one organ — your liver.Sugary drinks most common way to consume excessive, unneeded amounts of fructose.When you consume too much, your liver becomes overloaded which then converts the fructose into fat.Some of the fat gets shipped out as blood triglycerides, while part of it remains in your liver. Over time, this can contribute to nonalcoholic fatty liver disease. Sucrose and high-fructose corn syrup are about 50% fructose, which can only be metabolized by your liver. Excessive amounts may contribute to nonalcoholic fatty liver disease.

# 3. Sugar Drastically Increases Belly Fat Accumulation

High sugar intake is associated with weight gain. In particular, fructose is linked to a significant increase in the dangerous fat around your belly and organs. This is known as visceral fat or belly fat. Excessive belly fat is tied to an increased risk of type 2 diabetes and heart disease. In one 10-week study, 32 healthy people consumed beverages sweetened with either fructose or glucose. Those who consumed glucose had an increase in skin fat — which is not linked to metabolic disease — while those who consumed fructose saw their belly fat significantly increase. High consumption of fructose makes you accumulate belly fat, a dangerous type of fat linked to metabolic disease.

# 4. Sugary Soda May Cause Insulin Resistance — a Key Feature of Metabolic Syndrome

The hormone insulin drives glucose from your bloodstream into your cells. But when you drink sugary soda, your cells may become less sensitive or resistant to the effects of insulin. When this happens, your pancreas must make even more insulin to remove the glucose from your bloodstream — so insulin levels in your blood spike. This condition is known as insulin resistance. Insulin resistance is arguably the main driver behind metabolic syndrome — a stepping stone towards type 2 diabetes and heart disease. Animal studies demonstrate that excess fructose causes insulin resistance and chronically elevated insulin levels. One study in healthy, young men found that moderate intake of fructose increased insulin resistance in the liver. Excess fructose intake may lead to insulin resistance, the main abnormality in metabolic syndrome.

# 5. Sugar-Sweetened Beverages May Be the Leading Dietary Cause of Type 2 Diabetes

Type 2 diabetes is a common disease, affecting millions of people worldwide. It is characterized by elevated blood sugar due to insulin resistance or deficiency. Since excessive fructose intake may lead to insulin resistance, it is unsurprising that numerous studies link soda consumption to type 2 diabetes. In fact, drinking as little as one can of sugary soda per day has been consistently linked to an increased risk of type 2 diabetes. A recent study, which looked at sugar consumption and diabetes in 175 countries, showed that for every 150 calories of sugar per day — about 1 can of soda — the risk of type 2 diabetes increased by 1.1%. To put that in perspective, if the entire population of the United States added one can of soda to their daily diet, 3.6 million more people might get type 2 diabetes.A large body of evidence links added sugar consumption — particularly from sugar-sweetened beverages — to type 2 diabetes.

# 6. Sugary Soda Contains No Essential Nutrients — Just Sugar

Sugary soda contains virtually no essential nutrients — no vitamins, no minerals, and no fiber.It adds nothing to your diet except excessive amounts of added sugar and unnecessary calories. Sugary sodas contain little to no essential nutrients, only providing sugar and calories.

# 7. Sugar May Cause Leptin Resistance

Leptin is a hormone produced by your body's fat cells. It regulates the number of calories you eat and burn. Leptin levels change in response to both starvation and obesity, so it's often called the fullness or starvation hormone. Being resistant to this hormone's effects — referred to as leptin resistance — is now believed to be among the leading drivers of fat gain in humans. In fact, animal research links fructose intake to leptin resistance. In one study, rats became leptin resistant after being fed large amounts of fructose. Strikingly, when they reverted back to a sugar-free diet, leptin resistance disappeared. That said, human studies are needed. Animal trials suggest that a high-fructose diet can drive leptin resistance. Eliminating fructose may reverse the problem.

# 8. Soda IS Addictive

Soda is an addictive substance. In rats, sugar binging causes dopamine release in the brain, giving a feeling of pleasure. Binging on sugar may have similar effects in certain people, as your brain is hardwired to seek out activities that release dopamine. In fact, numerous studies suggest that sugar — and processed junk foods in general — affect your brain. For individuals predisposed toward addiction, sugar may cause reward-seeking behavior known as food addiction. Studies in rats demonstrate that sugar can be physically addictive. While addiction is harder to prove in humans, many people consume sugary drinks in a pattern typical for addictive, abusive substances. Sugary drinks have powerful effects on your brain's reward system, which may lead to addiction.

# 9. Sugary Beverages May Increase Heart Disease Risk

Sugar intake has long been linked to heart disease risk. It is well established that sugar-sweetened drinks increase risk factors for heart disease, including high blood sugar, blood triglycerides, and small, dense LDL particles. Recent human studies note a strong association between sugar intake and heart disease risk in all populations. One 20-year study in 40,000 men found that those who drank 1 sugary drink per day had a 20% higher risk of having — or dying from — a heart attack, compared to men who rarely consumed sugary drinks. Multiple studies have determined a strong link between sugary beverages and heart disease risk.

# 10. Soda Drinkers Have a Higher Risk of Cancer

Cancer tends to go hand-in-hand with other chronic diseases like obesity, type 2 diabetes, and heart disease.

For this reason, it is unsurprising to see that sugary drinks are frequently associated with an increased risk of cancer. One study in over 60,000 adults discovered that those who drank 2 or more sugary sodas per week were 87% more likely to develop pancreatic cancer than those who did not drink soda Another study on pancreatic cancer found a strong link in women — but not men. Postmenopausal women who drink a lot of sugary soda may also be at greater risk for endometrial cancer, or cancer of the inner lining of the uterus. What's more, sugar-sweetened beverage intake is linked to cancer recurrence and death in patients with colorectal cancer. Observational studies suggest that sugar-sweetened beverages are linked to an increased risk of cancer.

# 11. The Sugar and Acids in Soda Are a Disaster for Dental Health

It is a well-known fact that soda is bad for your teeth.Soda contains acids like phosphoric acid and carbonic acid. These acids create a highly acidic environment in your mouth, which makes your teeth vulnerable to decay. If you think deeper into that thought it makes your wonder if sugar can damage our hard teeth that what is it doing to our soft tissues, why are the many governments and "healthy organizations" supporting sugar? Food for thought.

While the acids in soda can themselves cause damage, it is the combination with sugar that makes soda particularly harmful. Sugar provides easily digestible energy for the bad bacteria in your mouth. This, combined with the acids, wreaks havoc on dental health over time.The acids in soda create an acidic environment in your mouth, while the sugar feeds the harmful bacteria that reside there. This can have severe adverse effects on dental health.

# 12. Soda Drinkers Have a Drastically Increased Risk of Gout

Gout is a medical condition characterized by inflammation and pain in your joints, particularly your big toes. Gout typically occurs when high levels of uric acid in the blood become crystallized. Fructose is the main carbohydrate known to increase uric acid levels Consequently, many large observational studies have determined strong links between sugar-sweetened drinks and gout. Moreover, long-term studies tie sugary soda to a 75% increased risk of gout in women and an almost 50% increased risk in men. People who frequently down sugary drinks appear to have an increased risk of gout.

# 13. Sugar Consumption Is Linked to an Increased Risk of Dementia

Dementia is a collective term for declines in brain function in older adults. The most common form is Alzheimer's disease. Research shows that any incremental increase in blood sugar is strongly associated with an increased risk of dementia. In other words, the higher your blood sugar, the higher your risk of dementia. Because sugar-sweetened beverages lead to rapid spikes in blood sugar, it makes sense that they could increase your risk of dementia.Rodent studies note that large doses of sugary drinks can impair memory and decision-making capabilities. Some studies indicate that high blood sugar levels raise your risk of dementia.

# The Bottom Line

Drinking high amounts of sugar-sweetened beverages — such as soda — can have various adverse impacts on your health. These range from increased chances of tooth decay to a higher risk of heart disease and metabolic disorders like type 2 diabetes. Regular consumption of sugary soda also appears to be a consistent risk factor for weight gain and obesity. If you want to lose weight, avoid chronic disease, and live longer, start by limiting or completely cutting out your intake of sugary drinks.

# *The Plan*

*For the first 1 or 2 weeks, this may be difficult for you. We are essentially shrinking our stomachs, and replacing bad habits with good habits all in one. Do not skip breakfast! I repeat Do Not Skip Breakfast. Remember, our body needs the fuel to carry on through the day to not feel tired, to be full.*

*I wake up every morning at 5 am. This is not necessary for you to do, it's just what my body clock is used to. When I get up, my water is waiting for me. 16oz of water to start the day. I do calisthenic exercises in the morning such as jumping jacks, situps or push ups to get my blood pumping at the start of the day and get my metabolism on the right track. Sometimes I run the treadmill or lift weights depending on the day.*

*I buy the cheap brands, and that includes my tea. I use my store brand of green tea or black tea. It is cheaper, and it doesn't make a difference.*

*I sit at my computer for a large part of the day, so while I am sitting there, taking a small break, I do my isometric exercises. Sometimes while I am working I do it. It depends on what part of the body I am working on. It is pretty difficult to work on your arm muscles while typing, so I have to take a break to do those, but the legs exercises are pretty easy to do.*

*2 avocados, 3 pieces of buttered toast and usually some vegan sausages for breakfast. MMHMM!. Depending on the day, sometimes I make guacamole, other days it is for avocado toast. If you can't handle the thought of avocados(it took me a while to get used to it), you can substitute it for oatmeal, cold cereal but nothing with sugar. Eggs are packed with protein and are also a good start for your day. The point here is to start off your day right, and have some kind of breakfast. If not, your body is in starvation mode, and therefore starts to store fat because it thinks you are trying to starve it. The body is wonderful that way. It is self-preservation at its best.*

*One thing I would like to add to this. I use real butter only. I did some research a few years back about the benefits of margarine for a healthier lifestyle. I was shocked to find out that margarine is actually only 1 molecule away from plastic. Your body gets confused with chemicals. The body knows how to break down butter...so I haven't touched margarine since.*

*2 to 3 hours after breakfast, grab yourself an apple, banana, a carrot, whatever you have that is fresh and wholesome. This is to satisfy any craving you may have at this point. It is not lunch so don't worry.*

*For lunch, I make myself something filling but not too heavy. A can of soup, normally water based, salad or maybe a piece of fish baked or air fried.  Don't get stuck giving yourself something that you can't tolerate. I sometimes treat myself with sushi or pizza(vegan) or a burrito bowl but not often. There's a lot of sugar in bread, but hey, that why it should only be a treat. Just don't go overboard or it will defeats the whole purpose.*

*If I get hungry again a couple of hours later, you guessed it, cashews. Make sure to stay hydrated throughout the day. It will cut down on the hunger pains throughout the day and it will cause you to eat less during your meals. Water is essential for the body. You will be surprised how much just having water to drink will help your weight loss, again i recommend water but there are times when you get tired of water if so i try green tea hot or cold, maybe ice tead.*

*Dinner time is at about 6 or 7pm. I have another cup of water about a half hour before mealtime. This helps raise my metabolic rate to where I am not as hungry as I had been in the past. (This is according to my research. I was curious to learn why I was dropping so much weight.) For the first 2 weeks I ate very little pasta, and no fried foods at all. Those are the only 2 things I gave up over the 2 week period. Instead, I would eat sensibly. I started off with a small salad with just a small amount of dressing, (just enough to flavor it slightly,) and some baked chicken or fish. It was satisfying for my taste buds, and I felt full. I no longer heaped my plate with mashed potatoes and gravy, or whatever the starch was that night. I just held off, and realized that it didn't need that much food to feel satisfied.  After dinner around 8 0r ( if i'm still hungry i will drink green tea to help subside the hunger pains( not real pains just your body has to get used to the way you are eating now).*

*After 2 weeks of eating this way, I was feeling better than I had in years. I had lost about 30 pounds during the first 2 weeks, and I was hungry for more. I didn't want to be fat any more, and knew that I had stumbled upon the solution to get me back into shape.*

*I was amazed at how simple it actually was. I was losing weight, and not suffering. I was eating pretty much what I had been before, only in smaller amounts, and I was happy. I decided to take it to the next level. My stomach either shrunk, or my metabolism changed, or something, but I no longer needed, nor did i want, vast amounts of food. I like the feeling of being comfortable.*

*Since all of this was making sense to me now, I continued down that same path. Only I missed my pizza so I started eating that again. I continued with my green tea, and ate half as much as I used to. As an example, before all this started, I would eat a whole pizza in one sitting. I still think I could if I tried, but why? I am very comfortable eating half, and saving the other half for my lunch the next day. I am full and that is what my body wants. My stomach doesn't want any more food, so why would I continue to stuff it? It would only make me feel miserable and reverse all the hard work I put in to lose the weight.*

*Instead of a plate mounded with spaghetti, I chose to eat half that amount. Again, because of the combination of green tea before dinner, and my smaller stomach, I didn't need any more than what I had dished up for myself. Many times I didn't even finish what I had in front of me. THAT is another problem. Ever heard this before? "The eyes are bigger than the stomach." We are taught from an early age to finish what is on our plates. If we follow that logic, we need to put less food on there in the first place. Don't let your taste buds tell you that you have to have more, when your stomach is telling you otherwise. It is not healthy, and you will eventually get back into the trap of forcing your stomach to grow again. Little by little, we will keep expanding our stomach to its former size and we don't want that to happen.*

*That is the only thing I did in my weight loss strategy, and I am continuing to lose weight as we speak. Continuing with my green tea, eating healthier without becoming fanatical about it, and at this point, eating what I want...only in smaller portions.*

*You may have noticed that I have not said anything about calories so far, so let's chat about that for a bit.*

*A calorie is a unit of energy. We will not go into the scientific speak to explain everything it is and does. Human beings need energy to survive to breathe, move, pump blood and they acquire this energy from food. The number of calories in a food is a measure of how much potential energy that food possesses. A gram of carbohydrates has 4 calories, a gram of protein has 4 calories and a gram of fat has 9 calories. Foods are a compilation of these three building blocks. So if you know how many carbohydrates, fats and proteins are in any given food, you know how many calories, or how much energy, that food contains.*

*It seems that every food in the grocery store has the amount of calories on the label. It seems that the normal intake of calories they figure for a person is about 2,000 calories per day. This varies from person to person, however. A lot depends on how active your lifestyle is. A person like me, (relatively inactive because I spend most days planted in front of a computer) needs less calories than an active person who slings heavy boxes all day long.*

*The chart below will give you a rough idea of how many calories you use in a day, according to your lifestyle.*

| POUNDS YOU WEIGH | RESTING CALORIES | LOW ACTIVITY | MEDIUM ACTIVITY | HIGH ACTIVITY |
|---|---|---|---|---|
| **100** | **1,120** | **1,450** | **1,570** | **1,680** |
| 110 | 1,150 | 1,490 | 1,600 | 1,720 |
| 120 | 1,190 | 1,550 | 1,670 | 1,780 |
| 130 | 1,220 | 1,580 | 1,700 | 1,830 |
| 140 | 1,250 | 1,630 | 1,750 | 1,880 |
| **150** | **1,280** | **1,660** | **1,800** | **1,920** |
| 160 | 1,320 | 1,720 | 1,850 | 1,980 |
| 170 | 1,350 | 1,750 | 1,890 | 2,000 |
| 180 | 1,380 | 1,790 | 1,930 | 2,070 |
| 190 | 1,420 | 1,850 | 1,990 | 2,100 |
| **200** | **1,450** | **1,880** | **2,030** | **2,180** |
| 210 | 1,480 | 1,950 | 2,050 | 2,200 |
| 220 | 1,512 | 1,970 | 2,100 | 2,270 |
| 230 | 1,540 | 2,000 | 2,160 | 2,300 |
| 240 | 1,580 | 2,050 | 2,200 | 2,400 |
| **250** | **1,610** | **2,090** | **2,250** | **2,410** |
| 260 | 1,640 | 2,130 | 2,300 | 2,460 |
| 270 | 1,676 | 2,170 | 2,350 | 2,500 |
| 280 | 1,710 | 2,220 | 2,400 | 2,560 |
| 290 | 1,740 | 2,260 | 2,440 | 2,600 |
| **300** | **1,770** | **2,480** | **2,500** | **2,660** |

Resting calories is exactly what it sounds like. Calories needed to sustain your normal bodily functions, for instance things like breathing, heart beating, eyes blinking, and so on. If you happen to be sick, the caloric intake would be more, to help stop the infection.

You would be "Low Activity" if you have a desk job, and don't move around much or exercise. "Medium Activity" would be a person who, even with a desk job, goes out and exercises a few times a week. The "High Activity" would be someone who has a strenuous job, is a sports enthusiast and loves to exercise.

The key here is, to take in less calories than we need in a given day, and use up the calories stored as fat on our bodies. With the green tea, this magnifies because our metabolism is higher, so we will burn it more quickly.

Now,let's get down to business and see what we are supposed to weigh, according to the healthy chart.

| WOMEN | | | | MEN | | | |
|---|---|---|---|---|---|---|---|
| **Height Ft. In.** | **Small** | **Frame Size Med.** | **Large** | **Height Ft. In.** | **Small** | **Frame Size Med.** | **Large** |
| 4'10" | 102-111 | 109-121 | 118-131 | 5'2" | 128-134 | 131-141 | 138-150 |
| 4'11" | 103-113 | 111-123 | 120-134 | 5'3" | 130-136 | 133-143 | 140-153 |
| 5'0" | 104-115 | 113-126 | 122-137 | 5'4" | 132-138 | 135-145 | 142-156 |
| 5'1" | 106-118 | 115-129 | 125-140 | 5'5" | 134-140 | 137-148 | 144-160 |
| 5'2" | 108-121 | 118-132 | 128-143 | 5'6" | 136-142 | 139-151 | 146-164 |
| 5'3" | 111-124 | 121-135 | 131-147 | 5'7" | 138-145 | 142-154 | 149-168 |
| 5'4" | 114-127 | 124-138 | 134-151 | 5'8" | 140-148 | 145-157 | 152-172 |
| 5'5" | 117-130 | 127-141 | 137-155 | 5'9" | 142-151 | 156-160 | 155-176 |
| 5'6" | 120-133 | 130-144 | 140-159 | 5'10" | 144-154 | 151-163 | 158-180 |
| 5'7" | 123-136 | 133-144 | 143-163 | 5'11" | 146-157 | 154-166 | 161-184 |
| 5'8" | 126-139 | 136-150 | 146-167 | 6'0" | 149-160 | 157-170 | 164-188 |
| 5'9" | 129-142 | 139-153 | 149-170 | 6'1" | 152-164 | 160-174 | 168-192 |
| 5'10" | 132-145 | 142-156 | 152-173 | 6'2" | 155-168 | 165-178 | 172-197 |
| 5'11" | 135-148 | 145-159 | 155-176 | 6'3" | 158-172 | 167-182 | 176-202 |
| 6'0" | 138-151 | 148-162 | 158-176 | 6'4" | 162-176 | 171-187 | 181-207 |

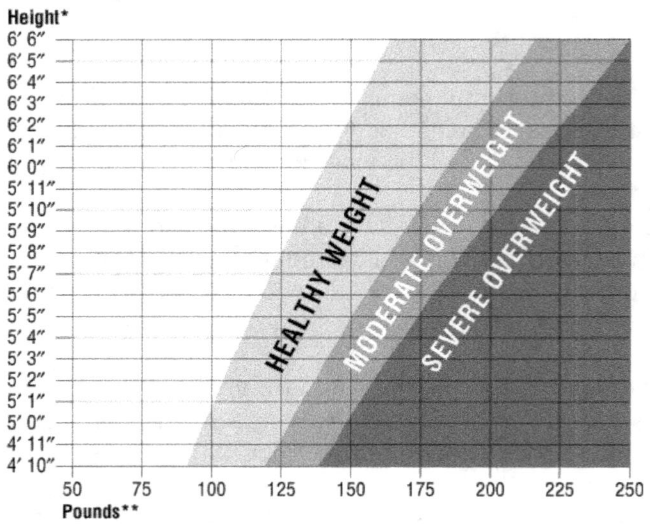


I could have made this guide much longer, but it was not necessary. My methods worked for me, and I believe they will work for you. I have made it short, and affordable so that everyone can buy it.

This is not brain surgery, although the weight loss "experts" may make you think it is. That is their way of doing it so they can hike the price up. I have given you all the information you need to lose weight and to lose it quickly. I will make a confession, through the holidays I did gain 4 pounds but I guess that is expected. I quickly shed those pounds in the next couple of days. I am now 230lbs my high school weight. I have never felt better.

If an inactive guy like me can lose that much weight, sitting in front of a computer screen, just think how much you could lose by following the methods outlined, and are a bit more active than I am.

I'm rooting for you!

J.C. Burns

www.ingramcontent.com/pod-product-compliance
Lightning Source LLC
Chambersburg PA
CBHW051729250726

48653CB00008B/3272